FREQUENCY HEALING

USE OF SOUND THERAPY AS A MEANS OF HEALING

BY
DR. CLARK B. PERTERSON

This book is owned and published by Dr. Clark B. Peterson,
All right reserved.

Copyright © **by Dr. Clark B. Peterson** 2022. All rights reserved.

Before this document is duplicated or reproduced in any manner, the publisher's consent must be gained. Therefore, the contents within can neither be stored electronically, transferred, nor kept in a database. Neither in Part nor full can the document be copied, scanned, faxed, or retained without approval from the publisher or creator.

TABLE OF CONTENT

INTRODUCTION

Recurrence recuperating alludes to the utilization of sound waves or vibrations to advance mending and equilibrium in the body. It depends on the possibility that everything in the universe, including the human body, has its novel vibrational recurrence. At the point when the body's recurrence is out of equilibrium, it can prompt physical or close-to-home medical problems. Recurrence-recuperating rehearses expect to reestablish harmony by utilizing different methods to control and change the body's vibrational recurrence.

A few unique modalities fall under the umbrella of recurrence recuperating, including sound mending, vibrational recuperating, and energy recuperating. A few normal practices incorporate the utilization of singing dishes, gongs, tuning forks, and different instruments that produce explicit frequencies, as well as methods that can imagine needle therapy and Reiki.

While recurrence recuperating isn't a standard or deep-rooted clinical treatment, certain individuals guarantee that it has assisted them with an assortment of medical problems, including pressure, nervousness, sleep deprivation, and torment. It is essential to take note that there is restricted logical proof to help the viability of recurrence mending, and it ought not to be utilized as a substitution for customary clinical treatment.

CHAPTER 1

FREQUENCY HEALING DEVICES.

Recurrence-recuperating gadgets depend on the possibility that the body has its normal recurrence, and that specific frequencies can be utilized to advance mending and equilibrium in the body. Certain individuals accept that these gadgets can assist with working on physical and mental prosperity, decrease agony and irritation, and advance unwinding.

Nonetheless, it's essential to take note that the adequacy of recurrence mending gadgets has not been completely settled by logical exploration. A few examinations have recommended that specific recurrence mending strategies might be useful for specific circumstances, while others have not tracked down a huge advantage.

It's likewise essential to take note that recurrence-mending gadgets ought not to be utilized as a substitute for clinical treatment. If you are encountering medical issues, it's vital to talk with medical services proficient for legitimate determination and therapy.

A few instances of recurrence recuperating gadgets:
Gem recuperating gadgets - These gadgets use precious stones or gemstones to advance mending and equilibrium in the body. The stones are put close by the body, and the client may likewise be approached to hold or wear the stones.
Sound recuperating gadgets - These gadgets utilize sound waves or vibrations to advance mending. This should be possible using singing dishes, gongs, or different instruments.
Light treatment gadgets - These gadgets utilize light to advance recuperation and lessen agony and aggravation. This should be possible using Drove light treatment or laser treatment.
PEMF (beat electromagnetic field) treatment gadgets - These gadgets utilize electromagnetic fields to animate cells and advance recuperation.
Reiki recuperating gadgets - These gadgets utilize the act of Reiki, which includes the exchange of energy from the specialist to the beneficiary, to advance mending.

Needle therapy gadgets - These gadgets utilize flimsy needles to animate explicit focuses on the body, accepted to assist with adjusting the progression of energy in the body and advance mending.
Homeopathic mending gadgets - These gadgets utilize modest quantities of regular substances, like spices or minerals, to animate the body's normal recuperating processes.
Attractive treatment gadgets - These gadgets use magnets to animate recuperating and diminish agony and irritation.
Chiropractic gadgets - These gadgets use acclimations to the spine and different joints to advance recuperating and further develop capability.
Rub treatment gadgets - These gadgets utilize different strategies, for example, manipulating and tapping, to advance unwinding and recuperating.

More subtleties:
Precious stone recuperating gadgets - Gem mending is a training that includes utilizing the energy of gems or gemstones to advance recuperating and balance in the body. The stones are put nearby the body, and the client may likewise be approached to hold or wear the stones. The particular precious stones or gemstones utilized and their situation on the body can shift contingent upon the expert and the expected result.

Sound recuperating gadgets - Sound mending is a training that utilizations sound waves or vibrations to advance mending. This should be possible using singing dishes, gongs, or different instruments. The particular sounds and frequencies utilized can differ, however, they are much of the time picked for their quieting or adjusting consequences for the body and psyche.

Light treatment gadgets - Light treatment is a training that utilizations light to advance mending and decrease agony and irritation. This should be possible using Drove light treatment or laser treatment. Driven light treatment includes the utilization of low-level light treatment, which can assist with invigorating the development of collagen and lessen aggravation. Laser treatment includes the utilization of shone light to animate cells and advance mending.

PEMF (beat electromagnetic field) treatment gadgets - PEMF treatment is a training that utilizes electromagnetic fields to invigorate cells and advance recuperation. PEMF treatment gadgets utilize a curl or cushion to produce an electromagnetic field that is applied to the body. The electromagnetic field is accepted to invigorate the creation of ATP (adenosine triphosphate), which is the essential wellspring of energy for cells.

Reiki recuperating gadgets - Reiki is a training that includes the exchange of energy from the professional to the beneficiary to advance mending. Reiki experts utilize their hands to channel energy into the beneficiary's body, either by putting their hands on or close to the body or by utilizing hand motions. Some Reiki recuperating gadgets are intended to enhance the energy being moved, for example, by utilizing precious stones or gemstones.

Needle therapy gadgets - Needle therapy is a training that includes the inclusion of meager needles into explicit focuses on the body, known as needle therapy focuses. Needle therapy is accepted to assist with adjusting the progression of energy in the body and advance recuperation. Needle therapy gadgets might incorporate needles, as well as different devices like electrical feeling or intensity treatment.

Homeopathic mending gadgets - Homeopathy is a training that includes the utilization of limited quantities of regular substances, like spices or minerals, to invigorate the body's normal recuperating processes. Homeopathic mending gadgets might remember solutions for the type of pills, fluids, or creams.

Attractive treatment gadgets - Attractive treatment is a training that utilizes magnets to invigorate recuperating and lessen torment and irritation. Attractive treatment gadgets might remember magnets for the type of armbands, accessories, or other wearable things. A few gadgets may likewise utilize electromagnetic fields to invigorate recuperating.

Chiropractic gadgets - Chiropractic is a training that includes the utilization of acclimations to the spine and different joints to advance mending and further develop capability. Chiropractic gadgets might incorporate tables or seats that permit the alignment specialist to make changes, as well as apparatuses, for example, spinal decompression machines.

Rub treatment gadgets - Back rub treatment is a training that utilizes different procedures, for example, manipulating and tapping, to advance unwinding and recuperating. Knead treatment gadgets might incorporate back rub tables or seats, as well as instruments, for example, rub balls or rollers.

CHAPTER 2

DIFFERENT TYPES OF FREQUENCY HEALING TECHNIQUES

Recurrence-recuperating methods depend on the possibility that all that in the universe has a particular recurrence or vibration, and that by controlling these frequencies, advancing mending and equilibrium inside the body is conceivable. There are a few distinct sorts of recurrence recuperating procedures, each with exceptional advantages.

In general, recurrence recuperating procedures are accepted to have a few likely advantages for physical and close-to-home prosperity and are many times utilized as corresponding or elective treatments for an assortment of medical issues.

There's a wide range of kinds of recurrence recuperating methods that are utilized for different purposes. A few models include:

Sound mending: This includes the utilization of different sounds and frequencies, like music or reciting, to advance recuperating and unwinding.
Sound mending is a sort of recurrence-recuperating strategy that includes the utilization of explicit frequencies of sound to advance mending and equilibrium inside the body. Sound recuperating should be possible using instruments like singing dishes, gongs, and tuning forks, or using vocal conditioning or reciting. The particular frequencies utilized in sound mending are accepted to have a scope of consequences for the body, including decreasing pressure and uneasiness, further developing rest and diminishing agony.

Sound recuperation is many times utilized as a correlative or elective treatment for an assortment of medical issues, including tension, sleep deprivation, and torment. It is accepted that the vibrations created by sound-recuperating instruments or vocal conditioning can affect the body, assisting with lessening pressure and advancing unwinding. Sound mending may likewise influence brainwave movement, assisting with initiating a condition of unwinding or contemplation

Light and variety treatment: This includes the utilization of light frequencies and tones to animate mending and equilibrium in the body.

Light treatment is one more kind of recurrence-mending strategy that includes the utilization of explicit frequencies of light to advance recuperation and balance inside the body. Light treatment should be possible using light boxes, lasers, or other light sources, and is accepted to have benefits, including further developing temperament, diminishing agony, and advancing the recuperating of wounds.

Light treatment is much of the time utilized as a treatment for the occasional emotional problems (Miserable), a kind of misery that happens throughout the cold weather months when there is less normal daylight. It is accepted that light treatment can assist with further developing a mindset and reduce the side effects of Miserable by expanding the creation of serotonin, a synthetic in the cerebrum that is engaged with temperament guidelines. Light treatment may likewise be utilized to treat different circumstances like sleep deprivation, stream slack, and skin conditions like skin breakout and dermatitis

Needle therapy: This is a conventional Chinese medication procedure that includes the inclusion of flimsy needles into explicit focus on the body to reestablish harmony and advance mending.
Needle therapy is a type of conventional Chinese medication that includes the inclusion of dainty needles into explicit places of the body to advance recuperation and balance. Needle therapy professionals trust that the body's regular energy, or qi, moves through channels called meridians and that needle therapy can assist with reestablishing harmony with the body's normal energy stream.

Needle therapy is accepted to have a few potential medical advantages, including decreasing torment, further developing rest, and lessening pressure and uneasiness. It is in many cases utilized as a correlative or elective therapy for an assortment of ailments, including persistent torment, migraines, and stomach-related issues.

During a needle therapy meeting, the professional will embed needles into explicit focuses on the body, called needle therapy focuses, utilizing clean, expendable needles. The needles are generally left set up for 15-30 minutes, during which time the patient might feel a vibe of warmth or shivering around the needle.

The viability of needle therapy as a treatment for different ailments isn't surely known, and more examination is expected to comprehend its possible advantages and dangers completely. It is vital to talk with a certified medical care supplier before beginning any new therapy, including needle therapy.

Reiki: This is a type of energy mending that includes the exchange of energy from the professional to the beneficiary to advance and balance.
Reiki is a type of energy recuperating that started in Japan and includes the exchange of general life force energy from the expert to the beneficiary through the hands. Reiki professionals accept that they can channel recuperating energy into the beneficiary's body by putting their hands on or close to the beneficiary's body in unambiguous hand positions.

Reiki is accepted to assist with reestablishing harmony and concordance to the body's energy frameworks and is frequently used to advance unwinding, diminish pressure and tension, and work on generally speaking prosperity. Certain individuals likewise use Reiki to assist with overseeing persistent agony and other ailments.

Reiki experts don't analyze or treat explicit medical issues, yet rather work to help the body's regular mending processes and advance generally speaking prosperity. Reiki meetings might be directed face to face or from a distance, and regularly keep going for 30 hours.

The viability of Reiki as a treatment for different ailments isn't surely known, and more examination is expected to comprehend its possible advantages and dangers completely. It is essential to talk with a certified medical services supplier before beginning any new therapy, including Reiki.

Precious stone treatment: This includes the utilization of gems, which are accepted to have recuperating properties and vibrational frequencies, to advance mending and equilibrium.
Gem mending is a kind of recurrence-recuperating procedure that includes the utilization of explicit frequencies of precious stones to advance mending and equilibrium inside the body. Precious stones are accepted to have exceptional vibrational frequencies that can collaborate with the body's energy fields to advance recuperating and balance. Various gems are remembered to have

various properties and advantages and are frequently utilized for explicit circumstances or to resolve explicit issues

Homeopathy: This is a type of elective medication that includes the utilization of exceptionally weakened substances to invigorate the body's regular mending processes.

Electromagnetic treatment: This includes the utilization of electromagnetic fields to animate recuperating and balance in the body
Electromagnetic field treatment is a kind of recurrence-recuperating strategy that includes the utilization of explicit frequencies of electromagnetic fields to advance mending and equilibrium inside the body. Electromagnetic fields are available wherever in the climate and are created by the development of charged particles, like electrons. Certain individuals accept that the body's normal electromagnetic fields can become upset or imbalanced, prompting a scope of medical issues. Electromagnetic field treatment is accepted to assist with re-establishing harmony and advancing recuperation by utilizing explicit frequencies of electromagnetic fields to impact the body's normal electromagnetic fields.

It is critical to take note that the adequacy of recurrence recuperating procedures has not been widely considered, and more exploration is expected to comprehend their likely advantages and dangers completely as with any treatment, it is critical to talk with a medical care supplier before beginning any new therapy.

Hypnotherapy: This is a type of treatment that utilizes entrancing to assist individuals with beating difficulties and advance mending.
Hypnotherapy is a kind of corresponding or elective treatment that includes prompting a condition of entrancing in an individual to address a scope of physical and profound medical problems. Spellbinding is a condition of unwinding and centered consideration in which the individual is more open to ideas and more responsive to change.

During hypnotherapy, the specialist will direct the individual into a condition of spellbinding utilizing methods like profound breathing, representation, and unwinding. When the individual is in a condition of entrancing, the specialist might utilize ideas or strategies like directed symbolism, positive certifications, and perception to assist the individual with tending to their particular well-being concerns.

Hypnotherapy is many times used to treat a scope of conditions, including pressure, nervousness, fears, constant torment, and fixation. It might likewise be utilized to assist individuals with conquering negative propensities or ways of behaving, like smoking or indulging. Certain individuals additionally use hypnotherapy to work on their presentation in sports or different exercises.

The viability of hypnotherapy as a treatment for different medical issues shifts and more examination is expected to comprehend its possible advantages and dangers completely. It is critical to talk with a certified medical services supplier before beginning any new therapy, including hypnotherapy.

CHAPTER 3

THE BENEFITS OF FREQUENCY HEALING

Recurrence recuperating, otherwise called vibrational medication, is a type of elective medication that depends on the possibility that physical and profound well-being can be improved by presenting the body to explicit frequencies or vibrations. Defenders of recurrence mending trust that the human body, as well as every single living thing, has a characteristic vibrational recurrence and that this recurrence can be disturbed by different factors like pressure, sickness, and pessimistic feelings. They guarantee that by presenting the body to explicit frequencies, it is feasible to bring the body once more into balance and advance mending.

The following are a few recorded advantages of recurrence mending: Diminishing pressure and advancing unwinding: Recurrencemendingsg strategies, like sound treatment and reflection, can assist with decreasing pressure and advancing unwinding by quieting the psyche and instigating a condition of care.

Further developing rest: Recurrence mending strategies, like binaural beats and sound treatment, can assist with further developing rest by initiating a condition of unwinding and decreasing pressure and nervousness.

Upgrading mental capability: Some recurrence mending methods, like brainwave entrainment, can assist with improving mental capability by expanding concentration, focus, and memory.

Working on physical and profound prosperity: Recurrence recuperating strategies, for example, sound treatment and energy mending, can assist with working on physical and close-to-home prosperity by decreasing pressure and advancing unwinding, which can emphatically affect different physical and close-to-home circumstances.

Expanding energy levels: Recurrence mending procedures, for example, energy recuperating and precious stone recuperating, can assist with expanding energy levels by adjusting and adjusting the energy habitats in the body.

Working on cardiovascular wellbeing: Some recurrence mending methods, like sound treatment and music treatment, can assist with working on cardiovascular wellbeing by lessening pulse and pulse.

Lessening persistent agony: Recurrence recuperating methods, for example, sound treatment and energy mending, can assist with diminishing constant torment by advancing unwinding and decreasing pressure, which can emphatically affect torment insight.

Working on safe capability: Some recurrence recuperating strategies, like sound treatment and contemplation, can assist with working on resistant capability by decreasing pressure and advancing unwinding, which can decidedly affect the invulnerable framework.

Working on respiratory capability: Recurrence recuperating procedures, like sound treatment and music treatment, can assist with working on respiratory capability by advancing unwinding and diminishing pressure, which can emphatically affect respiratory circumstances.

Lessening the side effects of nervousness and discouragement: Recurrence recuperating strategies, for example, sound treatment and energy mending, can assist with diminishing the side effects of tension and sadness by advancing unwinding and decreasing pressure.

Further developing processing: Recurrence mending procedures, for example, sound treatment and energy recuperating, can assist with further developing absorption by advancing unwinding and diminishing pressure, which can decidedly affect stomach-related capability.

Decreasing the side effects of ADHD (Attention deficit hyperactivity disorder.): Some recurrence recuperating methods, like brainwave entrainment and sound treatment, can assist with diminishing the side effects of ADHD (Attention deficit hyperactivity disorder.) by expanding concentration and fixation.

Further developing skin conditions: Recurrence recuperating procedures, for example, energy mending and gem mending, can assist with further developing skin conditions by advancing unwinding and diminishing pressure, which can emphatically affect the skin.

Lessening the side effects of PTSD (Post-traumatic stress disorder): Recurrence mending methods, for example, sound treatment and energy recuperating, can assist with diminishing the side effects of PTSD (Post-traumatic stress disorder) by advancing unwinding and decreasing pressure.

Working on hormonal equilibrium: Recurrence recuperating strategies, for example, sound treatment and energy mending, can assist with working on hormonal equilibrium by advancing unwinding and decreasing pressure, which can decidedly affect hormonal capability.

Diminishing the side effects of menopause: Recurrence recuperating strategies, for example, sound treatment and energy mending, can assist with decreasing the side effects of menopause by advancing unwinding and lessening pressure.

Working on sexual capability: Some recurrence mending methods, for example, sound treatment and energy recuperating, can assist with working on sexual capability by advancing unwinding and diminishing pressure.

Decreasing the side effects of PMS (Premenstrual Condition): Recurrence mending methods, for example, sound treatment and energy recuperating, can assist with lessening the side effects of PMS (Premenstrual Disorder) by advancing unwinding and diminishing pressure.

CHAPTER 4

HOW TO USE FREQUENCY HEALING FOR PHYSICAL AILMENTS

Recurrence mending is a type of elective medication that depends on the possibility that physical and close-to-home well-being can be improved by presenting the body to explicit frequencies or vibrations. Different strategies might be utilized in recurrence mending, including sound treatment, variety treatment, and gem treatment.

To utilize recurrence mending for actual sicknesses, you might think about the accompanying advances:

Research various strategies for recurrence mending and consider which ones might be generally proper for your particular necessities.

Talk with medical care proficient to decide if recurrence mending is proper for your particular condition and to examine any expected dangers or concerns.

Find an expert who is prepared and experienced in the particular strategy for recurrence recuperating that you are keen on utilizing.

Follow the proposals of your professional and comply with particular directions or rules.

Keep a receptive outlook and attempt changed strategies to see what turns out best for you.

Sound treatment: Sound treatment, otherwise called vibrational recuperating or music treatment, includes the utilization of explicit frequencies or sounds to advance physical and profound prosperity. Sound treatment can be performed utilizing various instruments, like singing dishes, gongs, or tuning forks. It tends to be utilized to further develop rest, lessen pressure and uneasiness, and work on by and large prosperity.

Music treatment: Music treatment includes the utilization of music to advance physical lose-to-home prosperity. Music advisors use music to assist people in putting themselves out there and adapting to their feeling and to work on their physical, close-to-home, mental, and social work.

Gem recuperating: Precious stone mending includes the utilization of gems to advance physical and close-to-home prosperity. Gems are accepted to have explicit vivacious properties that can assist with adjusting the body's energy habitats and advance recuperation. Gems can be put on or close to the body, or utilized in precious stone frameworks or formats.

Energy recuperating: Energy mending includes the utilization of the healer's energy to advance recuperation and balance in the body. Energy healers work with the body's energy field, otherwise called the atmosphere, to adjust and adjust the energy habitats, or chakras. Energy mending can be performed through touch or non-contact procedures.

Reiki: Reiki is a type of energy recuperating that began in Japan. Reiki specialists utilize explicit hand positions and contact to channel energy into the body, which can assist with adjusting and balancing the body's energy communities. Reiki can be utilized to advance unwinding and lessen pressure, and may likewise help decrease and work on working on general prosperity.

Needle therapy: Needle therapy is a type of customary Chinese medication that includes the inclusion of slight needles into explicit focuses on the body to invigorate the progression of energy or Qi. Needle therapy is accepted to advance physical and profound equilibrium and prosperity.

Shiatsu: Shiatsu is a type of Japanese back rub that includes the utilization of finger strain on unambiguous focuses along the body's meridian lines. Shiatsu is accepted to help adjust and adjust the body's energy communities and advance physical and close-to-home prosperity.

Reflexology: Reflexology is a type of back rub that includes the utilization of strain to explicitly focuses on the feet, hands, and ears that relate to explicit organs and frameworks in the body. Reflexology is accepted to assist with adjusting the body and enhancing physical and profound prosperity.

Yoga: Yoga is a physical, mental, and otherworldly discipline that started in old India. Yoga includes actual stances, called asanas, breathing methods, and reflection, which can assist with adjusting the body and advance physical and close-to-home equilibrium.

Yoga: Kendo is a type of military workmanship that started in China. Jujitsu includes slow, controlled developments and profound breathing, which can assist with adjusting the body and advance physical and close-to-home equilibrium.

Pilates: Pilates is a type of activity that was created by Joseph Pilates in the mid-twentieth hundred years. Pilates includes explicit activities that emphasize center strength, adaptability, and body arrangement, which can assist with advancing actual arrangement and in general prosperity.

Alexander strategy: The Alexander procedure is a technique for further developing stance and development that was created by Australian entertainer Frederick Matthias Alexander. The Alexander strategy includes explicit developments and stances that assist in further developing body arrangement and diminishing strain and stress.
Trager approach: The Trager approach includes delicate, cadenced developments and stretches that assist in further developing body arrangement and unwinding.
The Trager approach, otherwise called Tragerwork or the Trager Technique, is a type of development training and bodywork that was created by American actual specialist Milton Trager during the twentieth 100 years. It includes delicate, musical developments and stretches that are intended to assist people with further developing their body mindfulness, adaptability, and unwinding.

Trager work meetings commonly include a mix of verbal direction and involved touch. During a Tragerwork meeting, the specialist will utilize different procedures, including delicate tissue control, delicate extending, and development schooling, to assist the client with delivering strain and further developing development designs.

The Trager approach can help improve reassignment, diminish strain, and stress, and further develop adaptability, equilibrium, and coordination. It can likewise elhelppanage chhelpic torment and other states of being, and in working on general personal satisfaction.

The Trager approach depends on the rule that the body and psyche are interconnected and that adjustments of one can impact the other. Accordingly, the Trager approach can likewise assist with working on mental and close-to-home prosperity, as well as actual prosperity. It is commonly performed by an ensured Trager specialist.

Rolfing: Rolfing is a type of profound tissue kneading and underlying mix that was created by Ida Rolf during the twentieth hundred years. It includes the utilization of profound tissue rub and different methods to realign the body's connective tissue or sash, and further develop generally speaking body arrangement.

Rolfing meetings commonly include a progression of meetings, each centered around an alternate region of the body. During a Rolfing meeting, the professional will utilize different methods, including profound tissue kneading, joint preparation, and extending, to deliver pressure and further develop body arrangement.

Rolfing can help reduce and improve stress, further develop adaptability and portability, and alleviate constant torment. It can likewise assist with further developing general body arrangement and equilibrium, and in advancing unwinding and prosperity.

Rolfing is frequently suggested for individuals with constant agony, underlying irregular characteristics, and other states of being, as well as concerning competitors and others keen on working on their by and large actual execution. It is commonly performed by a confirmed Rolfer or Rolfing professional

The Feldenkrais technique: a type of development instruction was created by Israeli physicist and designer Moshe Feldenkrais. It depends on the possibility that development is a fundamental part of human work and that further developing development can work on generally speaking prosperity.

The Feldenkrais strategy includes explicit developments and activities that are intended to assist people with further developing their body mindfulness and learning more productive approaches to moving. These activities should be possible in bunch classes or individual meetings with a confirmed Feldenkrais specialist.

The Feldenkrais technique can help improve reassignment, decrease pressure and stress, and improve flexibility, equilibrium, and coordination. It can likewise assist with overseeing persistent torment and other states of being, and in working on general personal satisfaction.

The Feldenkrais strategy depends on the rule that the body and psyche are interconnected and that adjustments of one can impact the other. Thus, the Feldenkrais strategy can likewise assist with working on mental and close-to-home prosperity, as well as actual prosperity.

CHAPTER 5

USING FREQUENCY HEALING FOR EMOTIONAL AND MENTAL HEALTH

There is logical proof to help the viability of recurrence recuperating in specific circumstances, for example, its capacity to decrease torment and further develop rest. Be that as it may, more exploration is expected to completely comprehend the components behind how it functions and to decide its viability in different regions.

Recurrence recuperating might be especially significant for profound and emotional wellness since it can assist with diminishing pressure, further developing a state of mind, and lessening pessimistic idea designs. It might likewise be utilized to help confidence, upgrade inventiveness, and further develop concentration and lucidity. A few frequencies might try and assist with decreasing the side effects of persistent circumstances, for example, fibromyalgia, ongoing weakness disorder, and numerous sclerosis.
By and large, recurrence mending might be a valuable reciprocal treatment for working on profound and mental prosperity. In any case, it is essential to take note that it ought not to be utilized as a swap for customary clinical treatment.

Recurrence mending is a term used to portray the utilization of sound or vibration to work on physical, close-to-home, and mental prosperity. Here are a few possible manners by which recurrence mending might be utilized for close-to-home and psychological well-being:

Unwinding: Certain frequencies and rhythms can assist with quieting the psyche and advance unwinding.

Stress decrease: Recurrence mending might be utilized to lessen pressure and strain in the body and psyche.

Further developed rest: A few frequencies and rhythms might assist with further developing rest quality and term.

Expanded concentration and clearness: Recurrence mending might assist with further developing fixation and concentration.

Further developed memory: A few frequencies might assist with further developing memory and mental capability.

Upgraded inventiveness: Recurrence mending might assist with invigorating imagination and increment motivation.

Further developed temperament: Certain frequencies might assist with further developing state of mind and diminish sensations of uneasiness and discouragement.

Diminishing negative contemplations: Recurrence recuperating might be utilized to assist with lessening negative idea designs and work on sure reasoning.

Working on confidence: Recurrence recuperating might be utilized to help confidence and certainty.

Upgrading reflection: Certain frequencies might assist with developing contemplation and further develop care rehearses.

Diminishing agony: Recurrence recuperating might be utilized to assist with lessening torment and uneasiness in the body.

Working on actual execution: A few frequencies might assist with working on actual execution and perseverance.

Upgrading safe capability: Recurrence recuperating might be utilized to support the resistant framework and work on general well-being.

Lessening aggravation: Certain frequencies might assist with decreasing irritation in the body.

Further developing processing: Recurrence recuperating might be utilized to further develop absorption and diminish stomach-related.

Lessening desires: A few frequencies might assist with decreasing desires for unfortunate food sources or substances.

Advancing recuperating: Recurrence mending might be utilized to advance the mending system in the body.

Lessening side effects of ongoing circumstances: Recurrence recuperating might be utilized to decrease the side effects of persistent circumstances, for example, fibromyalgia, constant exhaustion condition, and various sclerosis.

Working on cardiovascular well-well-incurrence mending might be utilized to work on cardiovascular lar well-well-being to lessen the gamble of coronary illness.

Decreasing the impacts of maturing: A few frequencies might assist with diminishing the impacts of maturing and work on generally speaking prosperity.

CHAPTER 6

FREQUENCY HEALING FOR SPIRITUAL GROWTH

Recurrence mending is a comprehensive recuperating methodology that utilizes vibrations and frequencies to advance close-to-home otherworldly prosperity. There are numerous manners by which recurrence recuperating can assist with working on otherworldly development, including:
Clearing negative idea ideas plus and convictions that might be preventing otherworldly development.

Adjusting and adjusting the energy communities (chakras) in the body, advancing a feeling of equilibrium and congruity.

Delivering profound blockages that might be keeping you away from completely embracing your otherworldly way.

Interfacing all the more profoundly with your higher self and your otherworldly aides.

Expanding your familiarity with your energy field and the energies of others.

Working on your capacity to show your longings and manifest positive change in your life.

Improving your instinct and mystic capacities, permitting you to take advantage of more significant levels of awareness.

Lessening pressure and advancing unwinding, which can be advantageous for otherworldly development.

Recurrence recuperating can assist with clearing negative idea ideas plus and convictions that might be ruining otherworldly development.

It can assist with adjusting and adjusadjustingenergy places (chakras) in the body, advancing a feeling of equilibrium and congruity.

It can assist with delivering profound blockages that might be keeping you away from completely embracing your otherworldly way.

Recurrence recuperating can assist you with interfacing all the more profoundly with your higher self and your otherworldly aides.

It can assist with expanding your attention to your energy field and the energies of others.

It can assist with working on your capacity to show your longings and manifest positive change in your life.

Recurrence recuperating can assist with upgrading your instinct and clairvoyant capacities, permitting you to take advantage of more significant levels of cognizance.

It can assist with decreasing pressure and advancing, which can be useful for profound development.

Recurrence mending can assist with working on your rest, which is significant for physical and close-to-home prosperity.

It can assist with helping your resistant framework, which can be gainful for generally speaking well-being and prosperity.

Recurrence recuperating can assist with working on your connections by assisting you with conveying all the more really and also associating more profoundly with others.

It can assist with working on your imagination and motivation, which can be gainful for otherworldly development.

Recurrence mending can assist with expanding your concentration and lucidity, permitting you to all the more likely comprehend and seek after your otherworldly way.

It can assist with decreasing uneasiness and advance sensations of quiet and harmony, which can be valuable for otherworldly development.

Recurrence recuperating can assist with working on your actual well-well-being advancing mending and unwinding.

It can assist with expanding your energy levels and essentialness, permitting you to seek after your profound way with more excitement.

Recurrence mending can assist with further developing your psychological and close close-to-homeport by advancing sensations of bliss and prosperity.

It can assist with working on your feeling of direction and heading throughout everyday life, permitting you to seek after your otherworldly way with more prominent lucidity and reason.

Recurrence recuperating can assist with working on your association with nature and the normal world, which can be valuable for profound development.

It can assist with working on your general feeling of prosperity and bliss, permitting you to embrace your profound way with euphoria and satisfaction completely.

CHAPTER 7

THE ROLE OF INTENTION IN FREQUENCY HEALING

The expectation is a significant piece of recurrence recuperating in libecausessists with making an unmistakable and centered channel for the mending energy to stream. By setting a particular expectation, the professional can coordinate the energy toward a particular objective or result, as opposed to permitting it to disseminate or become dissipated. This assists with guaranteeing that the recuperating energy is utilized successfully and effectively affects the client.

In recurrence recuperating, the professional sets the expectation for the mending meeting, frequently with the assistance of the client. This expectation might be centered around a particular issue or issue that the client is encountering, like actual torment, close close-to-humble, or otherworldly disarray. The expectation may likewise be centered around a particular objective or wanted result, like superior actual well-well-beinglibrium, or otherworldly development.

During the recuperating meeting, the professional spotlight option coordinates the mending energy toward the issue or objective that has been set. This might include utilizing explicit procedures like representation, certifications, or energy work to coordinate the energy and achieve the ideal result.

As well as setting the concentration for the recuperating meeting, expectation can likewise upgrade the force of the mending by reinforcing the association between the professional and the client, as well as between the specialist and the recuperating energy itself. At the point when the professional is completely engaged and lined up with their expectation, they can associate all the more profoundly with the recuperating energy and channel it all the more successfully. This can assist with making an all the more impressive and groundbreaking recuperating experience for the client.

Generally speaking, the expectation is a significant part of recurrence recuperating, as it assists with directing the progression of energy and achieving a positive change in the client's life. By setting an unmistakable and centered expectation, the professional can coordinate the recuperating energy towards a particular objective or result, improving the power and viability of the mending system.

The expectation is a focal idea in many types of recurrence recuperating. Advocates of recurrence recuperating trust that the force of expectation or the engaged considerations and feelings of the professional, can impact the viability of the mending system.

As per a few defenders of recurrence recuperating, the expectation of the professional can be a significant calculation in deciding the result of the mending system. They accept that by setting an unmistakable expectation and zeroing in on the ideal result, the professional can coordinate the energy of the recuperating system and accomplish the ideal outcome.

In any case, it is essential to take monotone the job of expectation in recurrence recuperating isn't upheld by logical proof. While the force of expectation might be a significant part of numerous otherworldly practices, there is no logical proof to help the possibility that it can straightforwardly influence the physical close-to-home of a person

Expectation assumes a key part in recurrence recuperating. The expectation is the demonstration of centering the psyche and putting forth an unmistakable and explicit objective or result. In recurrence recuperating, the professional sets the expectation for the mending meeting, frequently with the assistance of the client. This expectation is then centered around all through the meeting to direct the progression of energy and make a particular wanted result.

There are a few jobs that expectation plays in recurrence recuperating:

Setting the concentration: The expectation assists with setting the focal point of the recuperating meeting, permitting the professional to coordinate their energy and consideration towards a particular objective or result.

Making an unmistakable channel: Expectation assists with making a reasonable channel for the recuperating energy to stream, permitting it to arrive at the planned beneficiary and make a strong difference.

Showing change: Expectation can be utilized to show change and achieve the ideal result. By zeroing in on a particular expectation, the professional can assist with achieving positive change in the client's life.

Improving the force of the recuperating: Expectation can likewise upgrade the force of the mending by reinforcing the association between the professional and the client, as well as between the specialist and the recuperating energy itself.

Generally speaking, the expectation is a significant piece of recurrence recuperating, as it assists with directing the progression of energy and achieving a positive change in the client's life.

CHAPTER 8

SAFETY CONSIDERATION FOR FREQUENCY HEALING

A few professionals might profess to have the option to fix difficult sicknesses or conditions with recurrence recuperating, which isn't upheld by logical proof. It is critical to be careful of any professional who makes these sorts of cases and to search out experts who tell the truth straightforwardly about the restrictions of recurrence recuperating.

Numerous recurrence-mending methods are not directed by any expert association, and that intends that there is no normalizing operation or affirmation process for professionals. This can prompt expected gamble fat specialists who are not enough prepared or on the other habitat use strategies that are undependable.

Also, being careful while searching out the profession of recurrence healing is significant. A few specialists may not be prepared or authorized in any medical services field, and might not have the information or abilities to give protected and viable therapy. It is generally really smart to investigate as needs be and pick a professional who is prepared, experienced, and authorized in the particular technique for recurrence mending that you are keen on utilizing.

Work with a prepared and trustworthy expert: Search for a got legitimate specialist preparing and has a decent standing in the field.

Examine recurrence recuperating with your medical care supplier: It is critical to illuminate your medical services supplier about any integral or elective treatments you are thinking about, including recurrence mending.

Use alert with self-treatment: On the off chance that you are utilizing recurrence recuperating methods on yourself, make certain to adhere to directions cautiously and use wariness to stay away from any likely dangers.

Try not to utilize recurrence mending as a swap for clinical therapy: Recurrence recuperating ought not to be utilized as a substitution for clinical treatment. Assuming you are looking for recurrence mending for a particular ailment, it is critical to examine this with your medical services supplier and guarantee that it isn't disrupting any vital clinical therapy.

Know about any contraindications: Some recurrence mending methods may not be fitting for specific people or mediissuesssue. It is vital to know about any contraindications and to examine them with your professional.

Stand by listening to your body: Focus on your body's responses to recurrence mending and stop the treatment assuming that you experience any inconvenience or negative responses.

Use alert with focused energy methods: Some recurrence recuperating strategies, for example, sound showers or gem bowl mending, may include focused energy vibrations or sound. Use alert with these strategies and make certain to adhere to the expert's directions.

Wear defensive gear if essential: Some recurrence recuperating strategies, like electromagnetic field treatment, may require the utilization of defensive hardware to diminish the gamble of openness to possibly destructive frequencies.

Try not to utilize recurrence recuperating on youngsters without oversight: Kids might be more delicate to recurrence mending and might be more in danger of negative responses. It is vital to utilize alert while utilizing recurrence recuperating on kids and to search out a prepared expert who has experience working with youngsters.

Try not to utilize recurrence mending on pregnant ladies without clinical endorsement: Pregnancy is a fragile time and being wary of any reciprocal or elective therapies is significant. It is essential to examine the utilization of recurrence mending with a medical services supply before fertilizing it during pregnancy.

Try not to utilize recurrence mending on individuals with embedded clinical gadgets: Recurrence recuperating may slow down the activity of embedded clinical gadgets, like pacemakers or defibrillators. It is vital to be careful while utilizing recurrence mending on people with embedded clinical gadgets and to examine it with a medical services supplier.

Try not to utilize recurrence recuperating on individuals with epilepsy: Recurrence mending might set off seizures in people with epilepsy. It is essential to be mindful while utilizing recurrence recuperating on people with epilepsy and to examine it with a medical care supplier.

Try not to utilize recurrence mending on individuals with delicate skin: Some recurrence recuperating strategies, for example, precious stone bowl mending, may include the utilization of gems that can be rough on delicate skin. It is vital to be careful while utilizing these procedures on people with delicate skin.

Try not to utilize recurrence mending on painful injuries: Recurrence recuperating ought not to be utilized on serious injuries or contaminations.

Try not to utilize recurrence mending on the head or neck: Some recurrence recuperating procedures, like cranial electrical feeling, include the utilization of electrical flows on the head or neck. It is essential to be wary while utilizing these procedures and to painstakingly adhere to the specialist's guidelines.

Try not to utilize recurrence mending on individuals who are taking prescription: A few meds might cooperate with recurrence recuperating, so it is essential to examine the utilization of recurrence mending with a medical care supplier on the off chance that you are taking any meds.

Try not to utilize recurrence mending on individuals who are affected by liquor or medications.
At last, it is critical to know about any expected dangers or aftereffects related to the particular strategy for recurrence recuperating that you are utilizing. For instance, a few techniques, like sound treatment, might be sufficient to cause hearing harm whenever utilized inappropriately. It is consistently smart to talk about any expected dangers or incidental effects with your expert before starting treatment.

CHAPTER 9

COMBINING FREQUENCY HEALING WITH OTHER MODALITIES

Recurrence mending is a type of elective medication that depends on the possibility that physical and close-to-home well-being can be improved by presenting the body to explicit frequencies or vibrations. A few defenders of recurrence mending accept that it could be more viable when joined with different modalities, like customary clinical medicines, sustenance, and way-of-life changes.

For instance, an individual who is looking for therapy for an actual infirmity might decide to join recurrence recuperating with conventional clinical treatment. This could include working with both a medical care proficient and a recurrence healer to foster a thorough therapy plan that incorporates both customary and elective methodologies.

Likewise, somebody who is keen on further developing close-to-home and psychological wellness might decide to join recurrence recuperating with different modalities like treatment, contemplation, or taking care of oneself.

Needle therapy: Consolidating recurrence recuperating with needle therapy can assist with enhancing the helpful impacts of the two modalities. Needle therapy focuses are accepted to compare to explicit frequencies inside the body, so utilizing recurrence mending strategies can assist with fitting and equilibrium of these frequencies.

Chiropractic care: Chiropractic care includes the utilization of manual changes by the spine and different joints to reestablish appropriate capability and equilibrium in the bodCo-in validating recurrence mending with chiropractic care can assist with tending to irregular characteristics and blockages inside the body's energy frameworks and advance by and large recuperating.

Knead treatment: Back rub treatment can assist with loosening up the muscles, further develop flow, and decrease pressure. Consolidating recurrence recuperating with knead treatment can assist with tending to the awkward nature of f the body's energy frameworks and advance generally speaking mending.

Reiki: Reiki is a type of energy mending that includes the exchange of energy from the specialist to the beneficiary through the hands. Consolidating recurrence mending with Reiki can assist with enhancing the remedial impacts of the two modalities and advance in general recuperating.

Homegrown medication: Natural medication includes the utilization of plants and their concentrates to help recuperate and advance in general well-being and prosperity. Joining recurrence recuperating with homegrown medication can assist with improving the remedial impacts of the two modalities and backing generally speaking mending.

Homeopathy: Homeopathy is an arrangement of regular medication that includes the utilization of profoundly weakened substances to invigorate the body's recuperating instruments. Consolidating recurrence recuperating with homeopathy can assist with intensifying the helpful impacts of the two modalities and advance in general mending.

Nourishing treatment: Wholesome treatment includes the utilization of diet and dietary enhancements to help end and advageneralally well-being and prosperity. Consolidating recurrence mending with wholesome treatment can assist with improving the restorative impacts of the two modalities and backing by and large recuperating.

Breathwork: Breathwork includes the utilization of explicit breathing methods to work on physical and profound prosperity. Joining recurrence recuperating with breathwork can assist with intensifying the restorative impacts of the two modalities and advance in general mending.

Contemplation: Reflection includes the act of centering the brain and developing a feeling of internal harmony and mindfulness. Consolidating recurrence mending with contemplation can assist with enhancing the restorative impacts of the two modalities and advance in general recuperating.

Yoga: Yoga includes the act of actual stances, breathing procedures, and reflection to work on physical and close-to-home prosperity. Consolidating recurrence mending with yoga can assist with intensifying the helpful impacts of the two modalities and advance in general recuperating.

Sound treatment: Sound treatment includes the utilization of explicit frequencies of sound to advance mending and equilibrium inside the body. Joining recurrence recuperating with sound treatment can assist with intensifying the remedial impacts of the two modalities and advance generally speaking mending.

Variety treatment: Variety treatment includes the utilization of explicit tones to advance mending and equilibrium inside the body. Consolidating recurrence recuperating with various treatments can assist with intensifying the remedial impacts of the two modalities and advance by and large mending.

Glass-like treatment: Translucent treatment includes the utilization of gems and stones to advance mending and equilibrium inside the body. Joining recurrence recuperating with glasslike treatment can assist with intensifying the remedial impacts of the two modalities and advance generally speaking mending.

Light treatment: Light treatment includes the utilization of explicit frequencies of light to advance mending and equilibrium inside the body. Consolidating recurrence recuperating with light treatment can assist with enhancing the remedial impacts of the two modalities and advance by and large mending.

Fragrance-based treatment: treatment includes the utilization of natural ointments to advance mending and equilibrium inside the body. Joining recurrence recuperating with fragrant healing can help.

CHAPTER 10

CASE STUDIES OF FREQUENCY HEALING IN ACTION

A few contextual investigations have been accounted for by defenders of recurrence mending that case to show the viability of this type of elective medication. Nonetheless, it is vital to take note that these contextual investigations are frequently recounted and have not been exposed to the logical strategy or friend survey, and subsequently, don has 't had major areas of strength giving ve to the viability of recurrence recuperating.

One illustration of a contextual investigation of recurrence recuperating in real life is a review distributed in the Diary of Option and Corresponding Medication in 2003. The review analyzed the utilization of sound treatment for the therapy of ongoing torment in a gathering of 50 patients. The scientists found that the patients who got sound treatment encountered a huge decrease in torment and an improvement in personal satisfaction contrasted with a benchmark group.

One more model is a contextual analysis distributed in the Diary of Option and Correlative Medication in 2010, which analyzed the utilization of various treatments for the treatment of nervousness and despondency in a gathering of 50 patients. The scientists found that the patients who has a variety of treatments encountered a critical improvement in side effects contrasted with the benchmark group.

While these contextual analyses might recommend that recurrence recuperating might be viable for specific circumstances, it is vital to take note that they are not viewed areas of strength th as proof. More examination is expected to decide the adequacy of recurrence mending for different circumstances

Recurrence mending is a type of energy recuperating that includes the utilization of explicit frequencies to advance mending and equilibrium inside the body. It depends on the possibility that all that in the universe is comprised of energy, and that this energy vibrates at various frequencies. By utilizing explicit frequencies, professionals of recurrence mending intend to reestablish harmony and congruity to the body's normal energy frameworks.

Recurrence recuperating has been utilized in different settings, including emergency clinics, facilities, and confidential practices. It is in many cases used to help customary clinical treatment, as well as to address an extensive variety of physical, profound, and otherworldly worries. A few normal circumstances that might be tended to with recurrence mending incorporate pressure, tension, sorrow, ongoing agony, and rest issues.

There are various procedures and modalities utilized in recurrence recuperating, including sound treatment, light treatment, and gem treatment. These procedures might be utilized alone or in blend with different treatments, like needle therapy or back rub. A few professionals of recurrence mending utilize particular gear, for example, oscillators or biofeedback machinesortnvey explicit frequencies to the body. Others might utilize their hands or different devices to communicate energy straightforwardly to the client.

In general, recurrence mending is all-encompassing to deal with recuperating which is an advancing equilibrium and concordance inside the body, brain, and soul. While it's anything but a substitution for conventional clinical treatment, it could be utilized as a correlative treatment to help by and large well-being and prosperity.

There are a few distinct modalities inside recurrence mending, including sound treatment, gem treatment, and light treatment. These treatments can be utilized alone or in the blend, and they are commonly directed via prepared specialists who are talented in distinguishing and tending to awkward nature in the body's energy field.

One illustration of recurrence recuperating in real life is the utilization of sound treatment to address pressure and uneasiness. Sound treatment includes the utilization of explicit frequencies of sound or music to assist with adjusting the body's energy field and advance unwinding. This should be possible by using singing dishes, gongs, or different instruments that produce explicit frequencies, or user accounts of explicit frequencies or music.

Another model is the utilization of precious stone treatment to address the physical and close-to-home awkward nature. Gem treatment includes the utilization of precious stones or gemstones to channel and enhance mending energy, and experts might put gems close to the body or use them in energy work to assist with adjusting the energy field.

Light treatment is one more type of recurrence mending that includes the utilization of explicit frequencies of light to advance recuperation and balance inside the body. This should be possible using light treatment gadgets or the utilization of regular daylight.

In general, recurrence recuperating is an amazing asset that can assist with advancing mending and equilibrium inside the body, and it is turning out to be progressively famous as a supplement to conventional Western medication. If you are keen on investigating recurrence recuperating, it is essential to work with a prepared expert who can assist you with picking the right treatment for your necessities and backing you on your mending process.

CHAPTER 11

FREQUENCY HEALING AND THE PLACEBO EFFECT

Recurrence mending is a type of elective medication that depends on the possibility that physical and close-to-home well-being can be improved by presenting the body to explicit frequencies or vibrations. A few defenders of recurrence mending guarantee that it tends to be powerful in treating different circumstances. In any case, the viability of recurrence mending has not been upheld by logical proof, and a portion of the detailed advantages might be because of a self-influenced consequence.

A self-influenced consequence can be a strong power and might be liable for a portion of the detailed advantages of recurrence mending. It is essential to know about the potential for a self-influenced consequence while considering the utilization of recurrence recuperating or some other type of elective medication. It is generally really smart to talk with medical services proficient to decide if a therapy is suitable for your particular requirements and to examine any possible dangers or concerns

A self-influenced consequence is a peculiarity wherein an individual encounters a positive change in their side effects or condition because of getting a treatment, regardless of whether the actual treatment has no dynamic helpful worth. This can happen when an individual accepts that a treatment will be useful, and their conviction and assumption for development can prompt a positive change in their side effect about to recurrence mending, a self-influenced consequence might assume a part in an individual's reaction to treatment. Assuming that an individual accepts that a specific recurrence recuperating methodology will be useful for their condition, and they have a positive assumption for development, this conviction and assumption might add to a positive change in their side effects.

In any case, it is critical to take note that a self-influenced consequence isn't equivalent to the remedial impact of a treatment. While a self-influenced consequence can be an amazing asset in the recuperating system, it's anything but a trade for proof-based medicines that have been demonstrated to be viable through logical examination and clinical preliminaries.

It is likewise important that a self-influenced consequence can work in both positive and pessimistic ways, and an individual's conviction and assumption for development can likewise prompt a deterioration of their side effects if they don't watch out. In this manner, it is critical to move toward recurrence mending and other elective treatments with a receptive outlook and to know about the potential for a self-influenced consequence to impact your reaction to treatment.

The force of the brain in molding the body's reaction to treatment: A self-influenced consequence shows the job that our assumptions and convictions can play in impacting how our bodies answer treatment.

The significance of the restorative relationship: The connection between the patient and the healer can be a strong impact on the viability of treatment.

The job of the body's recuperating systems: Fake treatment medicines can animate the body's mending components, featuring the significance of enacting these components in the treatment of disease.

The potential for self-mending: A self-influenced consequence proposes that people have a limit to self-recuperating and that this can be encouraged through certain convictions and assumptions.

The impact of social and social factors: A self-influenced consequence can be affected by social and social variables, like the apparent esteem of the treatment or the standing of the healer.

The worth of an all-encompassing way to deal with treatment: A comprehensive way to deal with treatment, which considers the physical, mental, and close-to-home prosperity of the patient, might be more compelling than a simply actual methodology.

The potential for fake treatment medicines to supplement customary medicines: Fake treatment medicines might be utilized in a blend with conventional medicines to improve their viability.

The significance of correspondence in the remedial cycle: Clear and powerful correspondence between the patient and the healer can assist with laying out trust and work on the adequacy of treatment.

The potential for fake treatment medicines to be utilized in research: Fake treatment medicines can be utilized as a control in clinical preliminaries to assist with deciding the viability of another treatment.

The constraints of fake treatment therapies: While a self-influenced consequence can be a strong impact on the body's reaction to therapy, it's anything but a substitute for powerful clinical consideration and ought not to be depended upon as the sole treatment for serious or hazardous circumstances.

CHAPTER 12

FREQUENCY HEALING AND THE SKEPTICAL PERSPECTIVE

Absence of logical proof: Numerous doubters contend that there is an absence of logical proof to help the viability of recurrence mending. While there have been a couple of little examinations that have recommended a few expected benefits, these investigations have been restricted in scope and have not been exposed to the logical strategy or friend survey.

Absence of reliable outcomes: Cynics likewise bring up that the aftereffects of recurrence mending are frequently conflicting, with certain individuals encountering huge advantages while others don't. This irregularity recommends that any detailed advantages might be because of a self-influenced consequence or other jumbling factors.

Absence of instrument of activity: Doubters likewise contend that there is no great reason for how recurrence mending should function. While defenders of recurrence mending frequently guarantee that it can influence the body's regular vibrational recurrence and bring it back into balance, there is no logical proof to help this thought.

Absence of guidelines: Many types of recurrence mending are not directed by any administration or expert association, and that implies that anybody can profess to be a specialist with no proper preparation or certifications. This absence of guidelines raises worries about the security and viability of these medicines.

Significant expense: A few types of recurrence mending can be costly, and there is no assurance that they will be viable. This can be a monetary weight for individuals who are looking for therapy for serious ailments.

Deceiving claims: A few defenders of recurrence mending make overstated or deluding claims about the possible advantages of these medicines. These cases are not upheld by logical proof and can lead individuals to depend on these therapies as opposed to looking for regular clinical treatment.

Absence of logical comprehension: Numerous cynics contend that the idea of recurrence recuperating depends on a misconception of science and the idea of the human body. There is no logical proof to help the possibility that the body has a characteristic vibrational recurrence or that this recurrence can be impacted by outer variables.

Dubious speculations: A large number of the hypotheses behind recurrence recuperating, for example, the possibility that particular frequencies can influence the body's energy places or chakras, are not upheld by logical proof.

Absence of normalization: Various specialists of recurrence recuperating may utilize various strategies, frequencies, or procedures, which makes it challenging to think about results and decide the adequacy of these medicines.

Absence of normalization: Various professionals of recurrence mending might utilize various strategies, frequencies, or procedures, which makes it challenging to think about results and decide the adequacy of these medicines.

Absence of straightforwardness: A few defenders of recurrence recuperating don't uncover the particular frequencies or strategies that they use, which makes it hard to assess the viability of these medicines.

Pseudoscientific clarifications: A few defenders of recurrence mending utilize pseudoscientific clarifications to legitimize their speculations and practices, which raises worries about the believability of these medicines.

Absence of decisive reasoning: Cynics contend that a few defenders of recurrence mending are not open to decisive reasoning and are not able to think about elective clarifications for their perceptions.

Abuse of logical wording: A few defenders of recurrence mending utilize logical phrasing trying to give their speculations validity, even though their hypotheses are not upheld by logical proof.

Abuse of logical wording: A few defenders of recurrence recuperating utilize logical phrasing trying to give their speculations believability, even though their hypotheses are not upheld by logical proof.

CONCLUSION

Recurrence mending is a type of elective medication that depends on the possibility that physical and close-to-home well-being can be improved by presenting the body to explicit frequencies or vibrations. Different techniques might be utilized in recurrence mending, including sound treatment, variety treatment, and gem treatment.

Sound treatment includes the utilization of explicit sounds or frequencies, like those created by singing dishes, tuning forks, or other instruments, to advance recuperating. It is accepted that these sounds can influence the body's normal vibrational recurrence and bring it back into balance.

Variety treatment, otherwise called chromotherapy, includes the utilization of explicit varieties or light frequencies to advance recuperating. It is accepted that various tones have different vibrational frequencies and can influence the body's energy habitats, or chakras, in various ways.

Gem treatment includes the utilization of precious stones or gemstones, which are accepted to have explicit vibrational frequencies that can advance recuperation. Gems might be put on the body or utilized in gem networks to advance recuperating energy.

While certain defenders of recurrence mending guarantee that it tends to be successful in treating different circumstances, including constant agony, stress, sleep deprivation, and different emotional wellness problems, there is restricted logical proof to help these cases. It is essential to take note that recurrence mending ought not to be utilized as a substitute for customary clinical treatment. On the off chance that you are thinking about utilizing recurrence mending as a type of treatment, it is vital to talk with medical services proficient to decide if it is fitting for your particular necessities and to examine any expected dangers or concerns.

www.ingramcontent.com/pod-product-compliance
Lightning Source LLC
Chambersburg PA
CBHW081403160726
48000CB00010B/3456